THE NEW HOMEMADE BODY SCRUB

The Easy and Quick Methods on Everything You Need To Know About Making Your Organic Body and Facial Scrub for Smooth, Soft and Youthful Skin

David Vogan

TABLE OF CONTENT

CHAPTER ONE

STEPS TO PREPARE SCRUBS

1. Coffee and Sugar Body Scrub For sparkling skin

You'll need

¼ cup ground espresso

¼ cup Sugar

2 tbsp greater Virgin Olive Oil

Three nutrition E drugs

Approach

Combine all of the elements until you get a rough paste.

Cleanse your pores and skin and apply this paste onto it.

Use your fingers to gently rub down the aggregate, in round motions, on your skin.

Take five-10 minutes to gently massage and exfoliate your body, spending 1-2 mins on every component.

Wash the aggregate off your frame with the use of hydrating body scrub and lukewarm water.

How frequently?

Use this body scrub approximately 2-three times per

week for an easy and sparkling skin.

The way it Works

That is one of the nice scrubs you may use for your pores and skin. Espresso is rich in antioxidants which help combat cellulite while the sugar on this aggregate works as an exfoliate that facilitates eliminate lifeless skin. The olive oil in this scrub penetrates deep into your skin, hydrating it and preserving it wholesome.

2. Sea Salts frame Scrub for glowing skin

Prep Time

Five minutes

Treatment Time

15 mins

Method

Combine all the ingredients until you get a coarse paste.

Cleanse your pores and skin and follow this paste onto it.

Use your fingers to softly rub-down the mixture, in circular motions, for your pores and skin.

Take 5-10 mins to gently massage and exfoliate your body, spending 1-2 mins on every element.

Wash the mixture off your frame with the use of a hydrating frame scrub and lukewarm water.

How often?

once every week for dry pores and skin, two times a week if you have normal pores and skin, and three times every week if you have oily skin.

The way it Works:

Sea salt is rich in minerals and exfoliating marketers that assist hold your pores and skin searching young and healthful. It helps improve blood circulate even as additionally reducing troubles along with scarring.

3. Coconut Oil frame Scrub for glowing pores and skin

You may need

¼ – ½ cup Granulated Sugar

½ cup Coconut Oil

Prep Time

2 minutes

Treatment Time

15 minutes

Method

Integrate the components till you get a coarse paste. Do now not warmth the oil as this could purpose the sugar to melt.

Cleanse your pores and skin and apply this paste onto it.

Use your hands to gently rub down the aggregate, in circular motions, to your pores and skin.

Take 5-10 minutes to gently rubdown and exfoliate your body, spending 1-2 mins on every part.

Wash the combination of using a hydrating body scrub and lukewarm water.

How often?

2-three times every week.

The way it Works:

This scrub isn't always the simplest and high-quality exfoliating agent, but it additionally allows cleanse your face, removes make-up, and moisturize. It's a notable finances-pleasant and smooth-to-put together remedy to be able to depart your pores and skin feeling like that of a goddess.

4. Olive Oil, Peppermint, And Sugar Scrub For glowing pores and skin

You may want

   ¼ cup Olive Oil

   1 cup Brown Sugar

   15 drops peppermint important oil

Prep Time

Five mins

Treatment Time

15 mins

Method

Integrate the substances till you get a coarse paste. Do not warmth the oil as this might cause the sugar to melt.

Cleanse your pores and skin and practice this paste onto it.

Use your hands to softly rub-down the combination, in

circular motions, on your pores and skin.

Take five-10 mins to softly rubdown and exfoliate your frame, spending 1-2 mins on each element.

Wash the combination off the usage of a hydrating frame scrub and lukewarm water.

How regularly?

2-3 instances every week.

How it Works:

This is a perfect tub scrub for the times that just don't appear to be happening. Enriched with the refreshing heady scent of peppermint critical oil, this bathtub scrub wakes and livens you up with strength.

5. Epsom Salt frame Scrub For sparkling pores and skin

You will need

1 cup Epsom Salt

2 drops of an important Oil Of Your choice

3 drops Jojoba oil

Prep Time

2 minutes

Treatment Time

15 mins

Method

Integrate the substances till you get a coarse paste.

Cleanse your skin and follow this paste onto it.

Use your palms to softly rub-down the aggregate, in round motions, to your pores and skin.

Take five-10 mins to softly rubdown and exfoliate your body, spending 1-2 mins on each component.

Wash the aggregate off your frame with the use of a hydrating frame scrub and lukewarm water.

How regularly?

As soon as a week for dry skin, twice every week for regular pores and skin, and three times per week for oily pores and skin.

The way it Works

Epsom salt is thought for its exfoliating residences and for how it enables smoothen difficult pores and skin. It's also claimed that the salt eases stress, relaxes your muscle mass, lowers blood pressure, and relieves soreness.

6. Oatmeal body Scrub for glowing pores and skin

You will need

½ cup raw Oatmeal

½ cup Brown Sugar

½ cup uncooked Honey

¼ cup Jojoba Oil

2 drops Lavender vital Oil

Four drops Geranium essential Oil

4 drops Frankincense

Prep Time

2 minutes

Remedy Time

10 – 15 minutes.

Technique

Grind the dry substances till you get a satisfactory powder and into it mix the liquid substances.

Combine the rest of the elements till you get a rough paste.

Cleanse your pores and skin and observe this paste onto it.

Use your palms to softly rub down the combination, in round motions, to your skin.

Take 5-10 mins to softly rub down and exfoliate your frame, spending 1-2 mins on every component.

Wash the aggregate off the use of a hydrating frame scrub and lukewarm water.

How frequently?

Twice a week

How it Works

Oatmeal is one of the pleasant herbal exfoliates. No longer only does it assists eliminate dead skin cells but it additionally soothes and heals pores and skin.

7. Yogurt frame Scrub for glowing pores and skin

You will want

1 tbsp Yogurt

¼ cup Olive Oil

1 tsp Honey

Three tbsp Granulated Sugar

Prep Time

2 mins

Treatment Time

10-15 mins

Approach

Integrate the components till you get a rough paste.

Cleanse your pores and skin and practice this paste onto it.

Use your arms to softly rub down the aggregate, in circular motions, for your pores and skin.

Take five-10 minutes to gently rubdown and exfoliate your body, spending 1-2 minutes on every element.

Wash the mixture off your frame the use of a hydrating frame scrub and lukewarm water.

How frequently?

2-3 instances per week.

How it Works

If you have dry skin however need to exfoliate regularly, this is the frame scrub for you. Yogurt has first-rate cleansing properties that assist easy your pores and skin with the aid of removing dead skin cells and impurities. It additionally helps moisturize your pores and skin.

8. Vanilla and Sugar frame Scrub for glowing pores and skin

You will need

1 ½ Brown Sugar

1 cup White Sugar

1 cup olive oil

1 tbsp pure Vanilla Extract

Prep Time

2 minutes

Treatment Time

10-15 minutes

Technique

Integrate the substances till you get a coarse paste.

Cleanse your pores and skin and practice this paste onto it.

Use your arms to gently rub down the aggregate, in round motions, for your pores and skin.

Take five-10 mins to softly rub down and exfoliate your frame, spending 1-2 minutes on each part.

Wash the aggregate off your body using a hydrating body scrub and lukewarm water.

How frequently?

2-three instances a week.

How it Works

This body scrub moisturizes your skin and keeps it searching younger and healthy. It correctly nourishes your skin and maintains it from getting broken.

9. Natural Turmeric body Scrub for sparkling skin

What you'll need

1 cup Sugar

2 tsp Turmeric Powder

1 ½ cup Coconut Oil

Prep Time

Five minutes

Remedy Time

10-15 minutes.

Technique

Integrate the elements till you get a coarse paste.

Cleanse your pores and skin and apply this paste onto it.

Use your hands to softly rubdown the mixture, in round motions, for your skin.

Take 5-10 mins to softly massage and exfoliate your body, spending 1-2 minutes on each element.

Wash the mixture off your body the usage of a hydrating frame scrub and lukewarm water.

How regularly?

2-3 instances a week.

The way it Works

Turmeric is one of the most famous herbal splendor substances used in India. It has robust antiseptic and antibacterial residences which assist preserve your pores and skin at its youngest fine.

10. Lemon and Sugar body Scrub

You'll want

2 tbsp Sugar

1 tbsp Honey

1 whole Lemon

Prep Time

Five mins

Treatment Time

10-15 minutes.

Method

Slice the lemon in half and squeeze its juice right into a bowl. To this, upload the opposite elements and mix nicely.

Cleanse your skin and practice this paste onto it.

Use your hands to gently massage the combination, in circular motions, in your pores and skin.

Take 5-10 mins to gently rubdown and exfoliate your frame, spending 1-2 minutes on every element.

Wash the combination of using a hydrating frame scrub and lukewarm water.

How regularly?

Two times every week

How it Works

Lemon is extraordinarily wealthy in vitamin C and allows give your skin a nourishment increase at the same time as also exfoliating it. It facilitates repair your skin's barely acidic pH stage even as ensuring that your pores and skin remains easy, gentle, and supple.

CHAPTER TWO

HOW TO USE BODY SCRUB

The usage of an exfoliating body scrub is a pretty clean undertaking to add to your pores and skin care routine. You just scoop a bit of the product out of the jar, observe mild pressure onto the pores and skin in a round movement, and then rinse off. On frame scrub days, avoid pairing with frame wash as using the merchandise concurrently regularly causes dryness. At the same time as the method of applying the product is straightforward, you do need to be aware of the following points in phrases of the way to exfoliate properly to avoid any headaches:

1. Ease the strain

Don't observe too much pressure when making use of the exfoliating body scrub to your pores and skin. Greater pressure does now not lead to higher gain. In case you sense any sort of ache, you will be eliminating wholesome tissue.

2. Temperature is important

Earlier than making use of the scrub in your frame, melt your skin with warm to warm water in advance. This can get your pores and skin prepared for exfoliation. If the water is too hot, you'll possibly become drying out your skin.

3. Experimentation

Feel unfastened to test. How to exfoliate differs for different humans relying on pores and skin kind and stage of sensitivity. If you have touchy pores and skin, start the usage of an exfoliating frame scrub first on a small patch of skin to peer how the body reacts.

Additionally, make sure to pick out substances wisely or you could boom your hazard of dryness or even breakouts. But don't worry too much! There's way more flexibility in the way to exfoliate your body overall as opposed to a way to exfoliate your face because the skin for your body is way less sensitive. One of the essential blessings of body scrubs is that you may attempt more than a few components you will be too hesitant to strive in your face. Test and have fun!

CHAPTER THREE

HOW OFTEN YOU SHOULD APPLY IT

As a widespread tenet, start off using body scrubs as soon as in line with week, after which gradually increase to three-four instances consistent with week. In case you are new to exfoliation, the first test on one part of your body. If you know you have got sensitive skin, communicate to your dermatologist first. Understand that absolutely everyone responds differently to exfoliation. Using an exfoliating frame scrub every day can worsen the pores and skin, even as exfoliating too sparingly received be effective, and you'll nevertheless turn out to be with the one's frustrating clogged pores and hardened skin that brought you right here within the first vicinity.

The advantages of frame scrubs received necessarily shine thru in all manufacturers. some frame scrubs use pretty harsh and abrasive substances, so make certain you select a logo or product this is obvious with its exfoliating components and makes use of gentle, plant-based totally components in its formulation.

CHAPTER FOUR

BENEFIT OF BODY SCRUB

1. An easy skin

An exfoliating body scrub works to clear away dry and lifeless pores and skin cells, leaving pores and skin refreshed, brightened, and oh so soft and clean. Just as you would on your face, why no longer supply your frame a few pampering too? Look for elements recognized for his or her pores and skin smoothing advantages, like sugar scrubs for frame exfoliation or different herbal sources of glycolic acid. Frame scrubs with sugar are fantastic for gentle exfoliation without irritation. Why not give your frame a facial?

With all the leaning, bustling, planking, and bending, elbows and knees tend to be the components of our pores and skin that want the most smoothing. Frustratingly so, elbows and knees also are generally the hardest components of the frame to smooth out, regardless of how plenty body lotion your practice. An exfoliating body scrub is frequently an excellent manner to smooth out those traumatic dry spots. Simply make sure to moisturize after exfoliation to fasten in the ones smoothing ingredients.

2. Moisturizer booster

Most beauty experts agree that making use of body lotion or dry frame oil after exfoliation accelerates the results of moisturizing. The hydrating and moisturizing increase happens due to the fact the exfoliating body scrub eliminates stupid and dead skin cells from your body, which lets in the pores and skin to take in creams greater simply and fluently.

An exfoliating body scrub can also be a notable addition to your acne-combating routine, as many body scrubs incorporate ingredients that help save you breakouts in your body by minimizing pores. Exfoliating with a body scrub also facilitates whilst making use of self-tanner for your pores and skin, supporting you achieves a glow without the streaks. Basic, the use of an exfoliating body scrub acts as a booster to assist maximizes the results of the products you follow to your pores and skin.

3. Razor bumps pores and skin comfort

Knowing the way to use frame scrubs before and after shaving can be an incredible way to calm and clean those frustrating razor bumps. Exfoliating with a body scrub, like our rose body scrub, can truly save you that stinging feel that so regularly plagues us after shaving! The skin clearing advantages don't cease here- frame scrubs additionally paintings to clean out rugged calluses, assist the arrival of dark spots, or even tame those devilish ingrown hairs post-shave or put up-wax by using pushing them up & out versus permitting them to curl under hardened pores and skin.

4. lengthy-lasting perfume

Past simply the pores and skin clearing benefits, the appeal of the frame scrub experience has loads to do with indulging in scrumptious fragrances. Basking in fragrant heaven is even easier with body scrubs as opposed to other pores and skincare merchandise due to the fact perfume has a tendency to last longer on exfoliated skin. Simply believe indulging in a cloud of Bulgarian rose oil after the use of a rose frame scrub infused with actual components. Now you can use your rose body scrub or sugar scrubs for frame exfoliation and take pleasure in this aromatic heaven all morning lengthy. An extended-lasting perfume, in particular, if derived from natural oils, will help soothe and loosen up your body and your mind as well. Now you already know why an exfoliating body scrub is frequently utilized in spa periods and massages.

5. Decompress & distress

Healthful pores and skin have both outside and inner effects. Exfoliating your frame's largest organ will actually depart you feeling rejuvenated. The little exfoliating beads of sugar scrubs for body exfoliation, as well as most other types of frame scrubs, will deliver your body the gentle rubdown it needs to strip away traumatic buildup, inside & out.

CHAPTER FIVE

WHAT YOU NEED TO MAKE A DIY BODY SCRUB

To make a DIY frame scrub, keep the subsequent items available:

Spoons for mixing

Blending bowl

Measuring spoons or cups

A carrier or base oil, inclusive of coconut oil, jojoba oil, grape seed oil, almond oil, or olive oil

Sealed field to store the scrub in

A few drops of your favorite essential oils, if favored

As soon as you have got the one's items, you can blend the oils with the granules of your desire, consisting of salt or sugar. You could also want to add other elements that could advantage your skin, like honey or inexperienced tea, as mentioned within the recipes below.

With self-made frame scrubs, it's vital to get the consistency proper. You don't want it to be too runny, which can make it hard to scoop into your arms, however, you furthermore might don't need it to be too crumbly.

Right here are some of the maximum popular kinds of DIY body scrubs that are both beneficial to your pores and skin and smooth to make.

Coffee scrub

There's some medical evidence that caffeine may additionally assist diminish the arrival of cellulite.

A 2011 study trusted source tested a cream containing

caffeine and other substances on 78 individuals. The study located that once 12 weeks of use, the contributors who used the cream noticed a full-size decrease in the appearance in their cellulite. A 2015 clinical study trusted supply related to 15 topics located similar results.

However, these creams contained other components, along with retinol, so it's hard to determine how powerful the caffeine is on its own at making cellulite less major.

That said, espresso is still a popular component for lots of DIY body scrubs. The tiny granules are gentle at the pores and skin, at the same time as nonetheless being powerful at putting off dead cells from the pores and skin's floor. And who can't withstand the aroma of a cup of espresso?

Elements

Half cup coffee grounds

2 tbsp. hot water

1 tbsp. coconut oil, warmed

Directions

Add the coffee grounds and hot water to a blending bowl. Blend thoroughly with a spoon.

Add the coconut oil. If needed, upload greater espresso grounds or greater oil to get the consistency right.

Whilst you're happy with the consistency, spoon the mixture right into a container.

Brown sugar scrub

Brown sugar is an inexpensive and handy ingredient that also does an awesome activity of exfoliating your skin.

Brown sugar is gentler on the skin than sea salt or Epsom salt. This makes it a perfect ingredient for touchy skin. The sugar granules may make your skin sense sticky, so make sure to rinse very well after you've exfoliated.

Elements

Half of cup brown sugar

Half cup oil of your desire, along with coconut, jojoba, olive, almond, or grape seed

Crucial oils (elective)

Instructions

Combine brown sugar and oil in a blending bowl.

Mix very well. If wanted, upload more sugar or oil to get the consistency right.

If preferred, upload one or two drops of your preferred essential oil, and stir it into the aggregate.

While you're happy with the consistency and perfume of your scrub, spoon it into a container.

Sea salt scrub

Salt has antibacterial residences that may be beneficial for some pores and skin conditions. Salt is also a preservative, so the sea salt scrub may be capable of naturally preserve itself.

Use ground sea salt, as coarse sea salt may be too harsh in your pores and skin. Sea salt scrubs can be too abrasive for touchy pores and skin. Additionally, be careful if you have a reduction on your skin because the salt can sting.

Due to the fact salt has no perfume; you could want to feature your favored critical oils to your DIY salt scrub.

Components

Half cup sea salt

Half of the cup oil of your choice

Critical oils (optionally available)

Directions

Integrate sea salt and oil in a blending bowl

Blend very well. If wished, add more salt or oil to get the consistency proper.

If favored, add one or drops of your favorite important oil and stir it into the combination.

When you're satisfied with the consistency and perfume of your scrub, spoon it into a box.

Green tea sugar scrub

Wealthy in antioxidants and anti-inflammatory homes, green tea may additionally gain your skin in numerous approaches.

Also, in step with a 2013 study trusted source, cosmetics that comprise inexperienced tea may be capable of reducing harm to the skin as a result of sun harm.

Inexperienced team can without difficulty is delivered to a homemade body scrub together with other nourishing ingredients.

Components

2 tea bags green tea

1/2 cup hot water

1 cup brown sugar

1/4 cup coconut oil, melted

Directions

Upload teabags to hot water. Let the tea steep until it cools.

While the tea is cooling, add brown sugar to a bowl.

Upload coconut oil and mix thoroughly with the sugar.

As soon as the tea has cooled, add it to the sugar blend. It's critical that the tea is cool so the sugar doesn't dissolve.

If the combination is simply too crumbly, upload greater coconut oil

If it's too soggy, upload more brown sugar.

Whilst you've reached the preferred consistency, spoon your scrub into a container.

Honey sugar scrub

Research trusted source indicates that honey has antibacterial houses. Consistent with a 2016 review trusted supply, honey additionally has antioxidant and antimicrobial Homes that may help an expansion of skin situations.

Not only can honey help restore skin tissue and protect in opposition to UV damage, but it can also assist kill germs on the skin.

Honey can without problems be combined with granules and oil to make pores and skin-nourishing frame scrub. After massaging the scrub into your skin, make sure to rinse your pores and skin off thoroughly to save you stickiness.

Ingredients

1/2 cup brown sugar

1/four cup coconut oil, melted

2 tbsp. honey

Instructions

Upload brown sugar, coconut oil, and honey to a mixing bowl.

Mix the elements very well, and upload extra coconut oil if it's too crumbly.

Once you've reached the preferred consistency, spoon your scrub right into a field.

CHAPTER SIX

SAFETY TIPS

These homemade scrubs are best meant to be used for your body, no longer your face. The pores and skin to your face are more sensitive than the skin at the relaxation of your body.

Keep away from exfoliating skin that is:

Sunburned

Chapped or damaged

Pink or swollen

Getting better from a chemical peel

If you need to add essential oils for your frame scrub, do a patch check with the diluted oil on your pores and skin first to ensure you're not allergic to the oil.

If you have touchy pores and skin or very dry skin, talk to your doctor or dermatologist to find out if exfoliation with a body scrub is right for you.

CHAPTER SEVEN

WHAT YOU SHOULD USE TO EXFOLIATE YOUR SKIN

There are extraordinary methods and equipment to exfoliate the skin. Facial scrubs and brushes are styles of mechanical, or physical, exfoliation. Acids and pores and skin peels are kinds of chemical exfoliation.

Mechanical

Exfoliating brush: This is usually a bristle brush used at the face or body to take away layers of useless pores and skin cells.

Some are designed for dry brushing. Others may be used together with your facial cleanser or body wash.

Exfoliation sponge: those are a gentler manner to exfoliate pores and skin. You could lather an exfoliating sponge with heat water, cleaning soap, or frame wash inside the bathe.

Exfoliating glove: if you locate brushes or sponges tough to grip, you can use a glove. Lather it with soap or frame wash in the shower. They may be effective for large areas including legs or arms.

Exfoliating scrub: this may be applied directly to the pores and skin with the use of a gentle, circular motion. You may wash your skin with heat water after making use of the scrub.

Chemical

Alpha-hydroxyl acids (AHAs) Examples of AHAs encompass glycolic, lactic, tartaric, and citric acids. Those work with the aid of breaking aside bonds protecting stupid and useless pores and skin cells to your skin's floor. This will reason your skin to certainly shed useless particles.

Beta-hydroxyl acids (BHAs) Examples of BHAs encompass beta hydroxyl and salicylic acid.

These may be higher for zits-susceptible pores and skin.